I0441833

Little Lupus Spirit Book:

Blending the Facts About Lupus With Spirit

by

Cory Hollingsworth

Certified Angel Therapy Practitioner®, Medium, Facilitator, Author

©Cory Hollingsworth WGA: December 2015

Cover Photo ©2016 "Zeus" - D.L. Weiss

I would like to dedicate this book to my fellow lupus Spirits.
You are blessed, loved, and supported during your journey.

I would also like to thank my family and friends for all of the love and support I
receive from you. Thank you mom, dad, grandma, and E. Ramírez (my amazing
child) for always being by my side.

With immense gratitude, I thank the Angels, Spirit, and my Higher Self for guiding
me to write this book and supporting me during the writing process.

TABLE OF CONTENTS

PART 3

"E-Motion" Steps and Affirmations from Angels and Spirit

PART 4

Breathing and Keeping Track of Stuff with Spirit as a Guide

Introduction

I am a Certified Angel Therapy Practitioner® and Spiritual Medium who lives with Systemic Lupus Erythematosis (SLE). Since my diagnosis with Lupus in 2011, my mission to guide others with their remembrance of Spirit has become an even stronger test of my personal faith in Spirit. Living with lupus is teaching me to be in a daily state of connection with Spirit and *acceptance* with lupus and its management.

I will be the first to admit that I am not *always* cheerful while managing my body and its condition with lupus. However, I have discovered that when this disease kicks me in the backside, I have the ability to remember my Spirit and manage this disease from a framework of empathy, compassion, self-care, acceptance, love, and light. I create and use affirmations and find ways to make my life simpler. I hope to share this framework with my fellow Lupus Spirits. I also wish to provide some easy and *practical ways* to manage lupus from the Love and Light of Spirit and the Angels.

I have done my best to keep the guidance in this book simple and "to the point" while maintaining the love and light of Spirit. The journey of Lupus can be paved with empathy, compassion, self-care, acceptance, love, and light.

PART 1: OVERVIEW

How It All Begins – Symptoms

The year 2011 was *very* bumpy for me. I began to miss several days of work and I became a constant presence at my doctor's office. Each time I walked into the exam room, I could almost hear the voice inside my doctor's head saying, "What now?" I had several discombobulated symptoms: persistent fever with no identifying cause, sudden weight gain and weight loss, extreme fatigue, weird rashes on my face, lesions on my hands and on my upper body, eye infections, and an overall sense of just not "feeling right".

One morning, after dropping off my son at school, I felt so fatigued that I parked my car at a nearby park and fell asleep – the fatigue was overwhelming. My body felt as if one more exertion could wipe me out completely. I appeared at my doctor's office the next day with a low-grade fever, swollen eyes, lesions in my mouth, and a very clearly defined rash across my cheeks and nose (known as a malar or "butterfly" rash). My doctor immediately referred me to a Dermatologist. Since lupus tends to mimic other diseases, lupus was not "the diagnosis" until everything else was ruled out. My Dermatologist biopsied and sutured almost every rash and lesion on my body. I began to refer to the procedures as "cookie cutter" moments. I reached a point when I would just surrender to my Dermatologist and say to myself, "Okay, here comes the cookie cutter." I was too tired to protest or get away (just driving to the doctor's office was overexerting for me).

After a couple of months of "cooking cutting", I received a diagnosis of Cutaneous, or Discoid, Lupus Erythematosis (DLE – skin lupus). I felt so relieved to have a diagnosis. My suffering and symptoms finally had a name. However, like most people, I had no idea what lupus was or what it meant to my life.

What is Lupus?

According to the Lupus Foundation of America™,

Lupus is a chronic, autoimmune disease that can damage any part of the body (skin, joints, and/or organs inside the body). Chronic means that the signs and symptoms tend to last longer than six weeks and often for many years.

In Lupus, something goes wrong with your immune system, which is the part of the body that fights off viruses, bacteria, and germs ("foreign invaders," like the flu). Normally our immune system produces proteins called antibodies that protect the body from these invaders. Autoimmune means your immune system cannot tell the difference between these foreign invaders and your body's healthy tissues ("auto" means "self") and creates autoantibodies that attack and destroy healthy tissue. These autoantibodies cause inflammation, pain, and damage in various parts of the body. Lupus is also a disease of flares (the symptoms worsen and you feel ill) and remissions (the symptoms improve and you feel better). Lupus can range from mild to life threatening and should always be treated by a doctor. With good medical care, most people with Lupus can lead a full life.[1]

---

[1] Lupus Foundation of America™ at lupus.org

The information I read about lupus from the Lupus Foundation of America™ (lupus.org) initially scared me. Apparently, my immune system was fighting *everything*. I imagined a large army of white blood cells going rogue and killing every cell in my body. No wonder my body always felt like it was in chaos. In addition, the realization that this disease could be life threatening frightened me. I assumed a diagnosis would enable me to experience some relief and function "normally" in my life. This is when I began to research my diagnosis with lupus.

Six Facts about Lupus from The Lupus Foundation of America™ Help Us Solve the Cruel Mystery™:

Fact 1) Lupus is a complex disease that is hard to define.

Fact 2) It strikes without warning, affects each person differently, and has no known causes or cure.

Fact 3) Lupus symptoms can be severe and highly unpredictable and can damage any organ or tissue, from the skin or joints to the heart or kidneys.

Fact 4) Living with Lupus can be baffling and isolating, as symptoms mimic other illnesses and often do not cause people to look sick.

Fact 5) While Lupus can be disabling and potentially fatal, in many cases the most serious health effects can be managed through aggressive medical treatment and lifestyle changes.

Fact 6) Awareness about Lupus among Americans of all ages is extremely low, with 61 percent of Americans reporting they have never heard of Lupus or know little or nothing about the disease beyond the name.

Source: The Lupus Foundation of America™ is launching the Help Us Solve the Cruel Mystery™[2] (lupus.org, 2014)

---

[2] http://www.lupus.org/page/-/files/pdf/Lupus_Factsheet.pdf

Find Resources – Learning About Lupus Helps Manage It

I am a natural researcher. I will read and dissect a topic of interest (or in this case, concern) until I am satisfied that I know everything about the topic. Lupus is an entirely atypical research project for me. Finding an all-encompassing source of information about lupus can be a challenge. The condition of lupus in and of itself is difficult to define, and the sources available to the layperson can seem overwhelming. Thanks to the Lupus Foundation of America™, I located another amazing source, *The Lupus Book: A Guide for Patients and Their Families* (2009) by Daniel J. Wallace, M.D. I quickly let go of my need to read *everything* about lupus and began to rely on the two amazing resources I had already discovered.

Fortunately, the Lupus Foundation of America™ and *The Lupus Book: A Guide for Patients and Their Families* (2009) answer most of my questions about lupus. Both sources also offer resources of their own (e.g., website links, further readings, teleconferences, etc.) that help me feel informed and comfortable with managing my life with lupus. I have also discovered a few books that have helped me with the emotional acceptance of lupus (see Works Cited and Recommended Reading). Find the resources that feel the best to you so you are able to answer your questions and concerns about lupus and manage your symptoms.

Doctors, Doctors, and more Doctors: Find doctors you like and who answer all of your questions

Once treatment began for my lupus, I began to feel a little better. I was able to function with more energy and vitality than I had during the previous year. I assumed that as long as lupus was limited to my skin, and stayed out of the systems in my overall body, I would be okay and I could just move on with my life. I assumed wrong. During the Spring of 2012, I began to feel the exhaustion again and, in addition, a new symptom appeared – the joints in my arms, hands, and feet began to feel painful and achy. I was accustomed to the achy feelings caused by the fevers of lupus, but these new symptoms began to sap my newfound energy and vitality. I told my Dermatologist about my new symptoms and she referred me to a Rheumatologist.

My first visit with my new Rheumatologist concluded with a diagnosis of Systemic Lupus Erythematosus (SLE). Lupus was officially in my entire body. I now needed to take lupus a lot more seriously. Of course, this new diagnosis meant more medical involvement with the management of my lupus. It also meant more invasive medications. I now had three doctors on my lupus team (with a couple of more added as time progressed).

I am very blessed to have an amazing team of doctors who guide me with treating and managing my life with lupus. It is important to find doctors you like and who answer all of your questions. The right doctors can make a world of difference in how you view and manage your symptoms and medications.

Spirit is Authentic: Beliefs and Thoughts

As an Angel Therapy Practitioner® who believes the body has the ability to heal itself, it is important for me to know the root *spiritual causes* for lupus. I often refer to one of my favorite books: *You Can Heal Your Life* by Louise L. Hay (2004)[3]. Louise Hay offers probable causes and affirmations (New Thought Patterns) for healing your body. According to *You Can Heal Your Life*, the probable Spiritual cause for Lupus (erythematosus) is: "A giving up. Better to die than stand up for one's self. Anger and punishment." (p. 184). At the time of my diagnosis, the affirmation (New Thought Pattern) of: "*I speak up for myself freely and easily. I claim my own power. I love and approve of myself. I am free and safe*" (p. 184), made little sense to me. Speaking up for myself and advocating my needs and wants were traits I always thought I possessed. However, lupus has become a catalyst for acknowledging I have some more speaking up to do.

"I Didn't Know Your Kind Got Sick"

Early in 2013, I finally began to disclose to clients and colleagues that I have lupus ("speaking up for myself"). Until that time, I would just tell inquisitive clients and colleagues that I was sick (a lot). One of my clearest memories of learning to *accept* lupus was when a client said, "I didn't think your kind got sick." My kind? I was not sure what "my kind" meant until I realized that many people believe that those of us who work in the Healing Arts (Psychics, Healers, Shamans, etc.) must live in a world where the body does not get sick, and when it does, we can magically make the illnesses disappear. I sometimes wish I could just wave a magic wand and make lupus disappear. However, I know deep down that my lessons with lupus are dynamic and include an important lesson with *Acceptance*.

---

[3] Hay, L. L. (2004). *You Can Heal Your Life*. Carlsbad, California, United States of America: Hay House, INC.

PART 2: The Lupus Spirit

Acceptance & Learning to Reprioritize:

Letting Go of Guilt and Redefining "Normal"

What is *Acceptance*? I continue to learn that one form of *Acceptance* stems from a knowingness that something exists that I may or may not have the ability to change…but I get to adapt for it anyway. I do not *like* lupus, but I *accept* that it is a part of my life and I need to adjust for it (daily).

A major component of lupus I am determined to *accept* is the concept of "normal". At the time of my diagnosis, I had a job, an additional part-time job at my church, played the role of single parent, and managed my sole-proprietorship as an Angel Therapy Practitioner®. My body was able to work six days a week in three alternating locations. I thought I could continue to maintain this pace of life in addition to managing lupus. I rarely asked my body what it needed. I would wake up, feel lousy, pretend my body was "normal", and move through my day as if struggling was an acceptable way of managing my lupus symptoms.

One Saturday, I awoke and discovered that I literally could not get out of bed. I was beyond fatigued. My body told me, "You are staying in bed!" I was planning to facilitate Angel Readings at a local store where I had been facilitating readings for almost five years. I felt an overwhelming sense of obligation to meet my clients and be present at the store. I fumbled out of bed and thought I could just "work through" the fatigue – it would "go away". Within about three minutes, I was calling the store to let them know I would not be making it in that day. I felt a simultaneous sense of guilt and relief. I had just taken the first step to redefining "normal".

During the next year, I resigned from my part-time job at my church and limited my time facilitating Angel Readings at the store. I began to focus my time and energy on my "day" job and my role as a single parent. I learned that reprioritizing my time and saying, "No" (mostly to my own feelings of guilt and obligation) enabled me to be present for *myself*. Saying, "No" also reaffirmed my power and my ability to speak up for myself (a New Thought Pattern: Hay, p. 184).[4]

Ask Your Body as a Friend, "What Do You Need?"

For most of us who live with chronic illnesses, our bodies frequently remind us of our limitations. Asking your body, "What do you need?" creates an energy of "What _can_ I do?" I have learned that asking my body what she needs for food, exercise, creativity, etc., has helped with most of my lupus symptoms. I feel like I am honoring my body as a friend by asking her what she needs, rather than focusing on her limitations.

---

[4] Hay, L. L. (2004). *You Can Heal Your Life.* Carlsbad, California, United States of America: Hay House, INC.

Find a way to pause and be still (quiet with deep breathing) and ask your body questions like: "What do you need to eat?", "Do you want to go for a walk today?", and "Do you need a nap?" The key to responding to these types of questions is to *follow through* with what your body tells you. If your body wants to eat kale, then eat kale (I like kale and it tastes even better blended into a smoothie with a frozen banana/fruit and soy/coconut/almond milk). If your body wants to go for a walk, then go for a walk (being mindful of when your body says, "Enough.").

Since the symptoms of lupus are unpredictable and can change from day to day, asking your body questions about *daily needs* can be a useful tool for understanding and accepting life with lupus. You will begin to focus on your *needs* rather than the limitations set forth by lupus.

Moving Lupus Facts into Spirit

Spirit Advice and Affirmations

The facts about Lupus can feel overwhelming and scary, so I decided to ask Spirit to guide me in offering some Spirit Advice and Affirmations. Affirmations are uplifting, positive phrases that can be read and repeated in an effort to create a sense of inner peace. When we examine each FACT about Lupus[5], and turn it toward Spirit Energy, we receive Spirit Advice that says:

Fact 1) Lupus is hard to define – Keep Explanations and Life Simple.

Since Lupus is "hard to define" by the medical field, it can even more difficult for those of us who live with lupus to define lupus for others. My job is to keep what I know

---

[5] http://www.**lupus.org**/page/-/files/pdf/Lupus_Factsheet.pdf

about lupus as simple as possible when I explain it for others. I usually tell people that my immune system attacks everything including healthy cells and tissue, and this causes inflammation in my body wherever, and whenever, it wants. Keep in mind: the average person probably does not want to know "everything" about lupus. Try to keep your life and explanations simple while keeping yourself informed about lupus. Even more important, keep your life and the "tasks" in your life simple.

Spirit says:

- **Keep life simple.** Be mindful of keeping your life simple so you and those around you avoid feeling overwhelmed. Let go of "the little things" that do not require immediate attention. Maintain the important things. Do what you can when you can. The "To Do" list may appear to accumulate, but overexerting and feeling stressed will only increase symptoms and fatigue. Find ways to make life simpler (discussed in more detail in Parts 3 & 4). .

Affirmation:

I let go of control and replace it with simplicity. I allow myself to do what I can in a manner that allows me to feel at ease. I am gentle with myself.

- **Take time to REST.** It is okay to rest and "do nothing". You continue to be an active member of the universe when your time is spent honoring your need to rest and take care of your body. No guilt. Your body requires extra rest and rejuvenation.

Affirmation:

My body needs time to rest and receive love. I send love and light to the parts of my body that are experiencing pain or discomfort. I feel safe knowing that my body is in full rest.

I use this "down time" to sleep, journal (digital recorders work great if writing is a challenge); listen to birds, read, and watch movies. I also spend more time meditating (or sleeping – whichever takes over first) and BEING rather than Doing. Nothing says you are required to be "doing" something all of the time – especially when your body is trying to heal and slow down.

Fact 2) Lupus affects each person differently - Be Honest about How You Feel and Make Sure Your Needs are Met

Each person who lives with lupus has a different experience. I have met people who are homebound and are not able to go out very often, as well as people who are in remission and are experiencing no symptoms of lupus. You get to learn what works best for YOU. Be completely honest with yourself, your doctors, friends, and family members. It is okay to describe every single symptom and medication side effect to your doctor(s). The more you express how lupus affects you, the better able you and your medical team are to manage it.

<u>**Spirit says:**</u>

- **Be Honest about How You Feel and Make Sure Your Needs are Met**

Asking for help is a sign of strength, not weakness. Prior to my diagnosis with lupus, I would have rather stumbled and fall than ask someone to help me with a simple task like opening a door, carrying a bag of groceries, or pouring water from a tea kettle.

12

I have learned that during my moments of pain and fatigue, it is wise to ask for help. As a result, my needs get met and I am honest about how I feel. You get to offer patience toward yourself and others and know that no one will truly understand what you need until you communicate your needs.

Affirmation:

It is safe for me to accept help from others. Being vulnerable offers another person and myself the ability to show compassion and strength. I accept compassion and strength as a sign of the unconditional love of Spirit. I accept offers of help with gratitude.

We are better able to focus on tasks that are more important when we allow others to help with the "little things" like opening doors, carrying groceries, and pouring water from a teakettle.

Fact 3) Lupus is Highly Unpredictable - Listen to Your Body: Be open to the ebbs and flows of life…and plan accordingly

One of the most annoying aspects of lupus is its unpredictability. One day, I feel like I am able to function effectively in the world, and the next, I feel like every inch of my body is frozen. In addition to the day-to-day unpredictability, we get to contend with the fact that lupus can strike any organ at any time. My lupus symptoms began with fatigue and skin rashes, but within a few months, my symptoms included my joints, my mouth, and hair loss. This level of unpredictability forces us to adopt a "living in the moment" lifestyle.

Spirit says:

- **Listen to Your Body: Surrender and be open to the ebbs and flows of life …and plan accordingly.**

Changing our routines to accommodate for lupus can seem challenging and wearisome. However, routine becomes vital to managing our symptoms. We still need to take medications on time, visit doctors and specialists, work, take care of a home, etc... I have discovered that the "unpredictability" becomes more acceptable when I listen to my body. I wake up, find out what my body needs, and then make a determination as to how my day will look: Am I going to work today? Do I rake the yard? Do I need to rest? Does the oil in my car really need servicing today? I listen to my body and plan the day accordingly.

I make a habit of keeping a large calendar in my kitchen with "important dates" (doctor appointments, workshop dates, special days, readings, etc.), so that I am better able to manage time. The *key* to maintaining a calendar is recognizing that sometimes events on my calendar *can change at a moment's notice.* I also schedule calendar reminder alarms on my phone to remind me when to take my medications throughout the day. It took about a year for me to let go of the guilt I experienced when I would miss work or need to reschedule an appointment. I have learned to surrender to the fact that my body will let me know what I am able to do during the day, and I need to follow through with what my body says. Surrender to the ebbs and flows…and plan accordingly.

Affirmation

I let go of external obligations that take me away from doing what is best for my body. I manage time day-by-day knowing that everything occurs in Divine Time. I can rest and relax knowing that the ebbs and flows of life allow me the opportunity to center my energies on being healthy and well.

Fact 4) Lupus often does not cause people to look sick- Express your needs and limitations to yourself and others

Those of us who live with Lupus do not always look sick. Most of us who live with lupus experience the majority of our major symptoms *inside* our bodies, so most people do not see lupus as a part of our presence. This fact has its **advantages** and **disadvantages**.

The advantage is that we do not usually look sick. It is usually not until my eyes (and/or face) swell that anyone even notices that I am sick. With the exception of those who know me well, or who worked with me prior to my diagnosis with lupus, no one would even suspect that I live with an illness that incapacitates me at regular intervals.

With the help of make-up, I am usually able to go to work and maintain a life outside my home without lupus "on me" and I am better able to "blend in" with everyone else. I can be camouflaged and "normal" looking to the world most of the time.

The disadvantage is that we do not usually look sick. Most people do not know that I am in pain most of the time, and I cannot be in the sun at all unless I want a rash and/or I want to sleep for three or more days due to sun exposure. I wear long sleeves and a wide-brimmed hat every day year-round (not exactly camouflage, but I am still able to appear somewhat "normal"). Most people assume that since we do not "look sick", we must be able to function at one hundred percent all of the time. This is when we get to remember our ability to *express our needs* to others. By expressing our needs, we do not overexert and add stress to our bodies.

Spirit says:

It does not matter if you "look sick" or not. Express your needs at all times.

I feel blessed to work in an environment where I am able to say, "I can't do that right now." I have been very up front and honest with the teacher I work with about my needs, and we have been able to make accommodations that allow me to instruct without feeling overwhelmed. The crucial factor is to tell others about your needs (and limitations) so that you and those around you are better able to understand and accommodate.

Affirmation

Others and I know my needs. I see the expression of my needs as an opportunity to be flexible and mindful about how I treat my body. I honor how my body feels despite the appearances of external or internal influences.

Fact 5) While lupus can be disabling and potentially fatal, in many cases the most serious health effects can be managed through aggressive medical treatment and lifestyle changes

Prior to my lupus diagnosis, I was (mostly) anti-Western Medicine. Most of my medical ails were treated with alternative methods such as herbs, homeopathy, sound healing, and meditation. When I began to take what I considered at the time to be "toxic medications", I was still in a state of denial that lupus would be a lifelong condition for me. Granted, the medications were helping my symptoms and enabling me to function in the world, but I still had an emotional and spiritual discontent for the medications themselves.

In my mind, I knew Western medication was aggressive, but it afforded me the opportunity to manage and maintain my daily life with fewer limitations from lupus. I have learned to accept my medications as <u>Light</u> rather than as toxins. I continue to use alternative/complementary methods (herbs, meditation, sound healing, etc.) with the acceptance that every medicine, herb, meditation, etc. is <u>Light</u> and blesses me with the ability to manage lupus.

<u>Spirit says</u>:

- **Get Rid of Negative Thoughts about "Aggressive" Medical Treatments**

I learned this technique from a colleague of mine, Marlene O'Neill. Each time I hold a bottle of medication (especially Prednisone®), I envision the bottle and its contents saturated in White Light (or any other color that seems suitable). I envision any of my perceived negativity toward the medication as <u>Light</u>. Each time I take out a pill and place it into one of my four daily medication reminder containers, I envision the pill being a <u>Light</u>. Each time I take my pills, I envision them as <u>Light</u> infusing into my body. If you are experiencing the process of injections or infusions, the same process of envisioning the medications as Light is just as effective as envisioning pills as <u>Light</u>.

Envision medications entering your body as liquid <u>Light</u> as you accept their abilities to heal. If you are experiencing dialysis, or a similar process, envision this process as a circulating Light entering your body.

This process of consistently envisioning medications as <u>Light</u> enables us to remember an *acceptance* of lupus rather than any negative perceptions. Try not to allow any negative thoughts or motives sabotage what your body requires of you in order to survive and thrive.

Affirmation

I honor my body and its individual needs. I am mindful about my feelings and conceptions about the treatments and methods that allow my body to thrive. I envision my body as a Being of Light and I envision any treatments that enter my body as Light.

Fact 6) 61 percent of Americans reporting said they have never heard of Lupus or know little or nothing about the disease beyond the name - Be an advocate for yourself (a New Thought Pattern, Hay (2004)).

I will admit that I was among the 61 percent of Americans who had never heard of Systemic Lupus Erythematosis (SLE). I am pretty sure Lupus was a disease I had heard "mentioned" at some point, but I had no idea what lupus was until I was diagnosed. According to Dr. Wallace (2009),

In the United States, nearly one million people suffer from lupus. It is more common than better known disorders such as leukemia, multiple sclerosis, cystic fibrosis, and muscular dystrophy combined. Those who develop SLE do so in the prime of life. And 90 percent of these sufferers are women, 90 percent of whom are in their childbearing years. Moreover, the effects of the disease disrupt family life and account for billions of dollars in lost work productivity (Wallace, 4)[6].

I find it staggering to learn that Lupus is more common than better-known disorders, yet we have very little knowledge of its existence. In addition: "In the United States African Americans, Latinos, and Asians have a greater incidence of SLE than Caucasians" (Wallace, 12). I may be going out on a limb to suggest that lupus receives little attention in the United States due to the gender and race of the people who live with it. I imagine that if lupus affected mostly Caucasian males, more effort to educate people about lupus and find a cure would be available. After all, I have heard of Erectile Dysfunction and Viagra® much more frequently in national media than I have about lupus.

Spirit says:

- **Be an advocate**

Be an advocate when you have the time and energy. Contribute when you can. One way I advocate for lupus is by joining the Walk to End Lupus Now®. I have yet to attend the Walk to End Lupus Now® due to time, fatigue, or illness, but I do my best to raise funds in its efforts. My Angel Therapy Practitioner® website has a link to the Lupus

---

[6] Wallace, D.J. (2009). *The Lupus Book: A Guide for Patients and Their Families*: Fourth Edition.

Foundation of America's™ website (and a link to this book as well). My goal is to raise awareness to the best of my abilities. Fortunately, due to social media, the word about lupus is becoming more common. If it feels right, share information from lupus-related websites and pages on social media. You are being an advocate by spreading the word.

A short time after my diagnosis with lupus, I wrote a letter to my family and close friends in an effort to inform them about my life with lupus. I included facts about lupus and the medications I was taking (and their side effects). I also included a statement apologizing ahead of time for missing any future family functions or events due to lupus flare-ups or fatigue. I figured the more my family and friends knew about lupus, the better able they would be to understand my needs. Those of us who live with lupus get to be *our own* advocates and spread the word (even if the word spreads only to family members and friends).

Affirmation

I advocate for others and myself to the best of my abilities. I allow others to ask questions while I offer simple insights and information. I emphasize the importance of learning about lupus and its effects on those who live with lupus.

- **Be Informed**

Nothing eases me more than knowing as much as I can about lupus. I do not always have the time or energy to appease my "natural researcher", but I have found it useful to peruse through the lupus.org website and follow links and websites that are of interest or importance to me. I also use *The Lupus Book: A Guide for Patients and Their Families* (2009) to find answers to my pressing medical questions and concerns.

Affirmation:

I allow myself to be a resource of knowledge for others and myself. I offer knowledge to others and myself about my life with lupus.

PART 3

"E-Motion" Steps and Affirmations from Angels and Spirit

As a Certified Angel Therapy Practitioner®, I work a lot with the Angels and other Spirit Guides to manage lupus. I call the messages I receive from the Angels and Spirit as "E-Motion" Steps. The Angels offer unconditional love and light to guide us into "motion" when we experience obstacles with self-acceptance. We learn lessons in empathy, compassion, and self-care. Choose the Spiritual affiliation that works best for you and ask for guidance.

Who are the Angels?

According to *The Angel Therapy Handbook* (Virtue, 2011), "An 'angel', in our terms, is a celestial (nonphysical) being who is an egoless messenger of God. In fact, the word *angel* derives from the Greek and translates to the phrase 'messenger of God.' Angels are deliverers of Heaven's love and guidance. Every person has at least two guardian angels. Your guardian angels are with you every moment of every day. They unconditionally love you, no matter what, and want the best for you. They never tire of you or get bored, frustrated, or upset with you (3-4).[7]

The Angels offer the following Affirmations and "E-Motion" Steps in loving guidance. Feel and use the messages that work best for you.

- **Self-Love**

Self-Love can be at an all-time low for those of us who live with lupus and other chronic illnesses. Even when others say, "You don't look sick," or, "You look fine", we know our bodies feel and act differently during our flares with lupus. We get to live with lupus *and* the side effects of the medications in our treatment and management of lupus (e.g., weight gain, moon face, acne, hair loss, ulcers, fatigue, skin rashes, pain, etc.). During this process, we also get to learn lessons of self-love and empathy (for others and *ourselves*).

My most dominant "self-conscious" feelings come from the weight gain I have experienced due to the side effects of medication. People who have not seen me for a while will say, "I didn't recognize you at first," or, they take a moment to look at me before they recognize me and say something. I understand my change in appearance can baffle some people (including myself sometimes) and this causes me to feel self-conscious in the moment. However, most of the time, the conversation usually moves forward with the fact that I am still "me".

---

[7] Virtue, D. (2011). *The Angel Therapy Handbook.* Hay House, Inc.

I continue to learn that my health is more important than my physical appearance (i.e., the side effects of lupus and medications). This is not to suggest that I no longer take pride in my appearance. It means that I am learning to accept and love myself *unconditionally* despite the outward appearances of my body. This body is mine and I get to take care of it and treasure it no matter what. I am discovering the more I love my body, the healthier I feel and the more energy I have. New Thought Pattern: "I love and approve of myself" (Hay, 184).

"E-Motion" Step – Radiate from Within:

Take some time LOOK at your body. Examine each arm, leg, foot, eye, toe, fingernail, etc. as if you are seeing it for the first time. Offer each part of your body unconditional love and support. Imagine each of your organs (kidneys, heart, lungs, brain, skin, etc) as strong and healthy. Offer each organ love and support. Envision your body as an ultimately strong and beautiful physical being.

Affirmation from Angels and Spirit:

My body is but one beautiful aspect of my true Divine Being. My power comes from within my Soul. I show others my Soul – the Light that is ME. When I radiate from my Soul, I radiate Love. I show others, including myself, LOVE.

"E-Motion" Step – Focus on YOUR Intentions and Make Time for You:

- **Make time for YOU**

Most of us lead active lives that center around the needs and wants of others. This small task will allow YOU to focus on YOUR intentions from the physical, emotional, mental, and spiritual aspects of your being. (note: You will need paper and a pen/pencil).

Take a moment (usually about a half an hour, or so) and BE in just YOUR energy. Find a room, close the door, and BE in your own space and energy without external distractions (e.g., cell phone, television, people, etc.). Write down your intentions for each aspect of your BEING. For example:

Physical: I intend to make sure I get more sleep.

Emotional: I intend to cry when I need to cry rather than hold in my tears.

Mental: I intend to read a book or write in a journal for fun.

Spiritual: I intend to spend more time in peaceful silence with myself.

Call upon the Angels and Your Higher Self (your Soul), to assist you during this process. Writing down your intentions will place them into the visual parts of your brain. This will activate a physical connection between your brain and your intentions, and allow you to "see" your intentions rather than just think about them. Do not worry if your intentions focus on only one or two aspects of your being (e.g., physical and emotional). Over time, your intentions will grow to include the physical, mental, emotional, and spiritual parts of your being. There is also no such thing as having "too many" intentions.

Just be mindful of creating and honoring the space and time you need to focus on a one (or a few) intentions at a time.

Once you have completed writing your intentions, take a few moments to look at your intentions and write down the "first step" toward fulfilling each intention. Ask the Angels and your Higher Self for guidance about creating the "first step". For example:

Physical: I intend to make sure I get more sleep. First step: go to bed at an earlier time and make sure that the hour prior to going to bed is free from distractions that prevent me from sleeping (electronics, television, chores). Listen to soothing music or sounds (or silence)- this can help calm my brain and place it into a state of rest.

Emotional: I intend to cry when I need to cry rather than hold in my tears. First step: Cry and not hold back – let it flow as a way to release. Find a trigger (like watching a movie that causes me to cry) if I feel the need to cry and am unable to let it out.

Mental: I intend to read a book or write in a journal for fun. First step: sit quietly with a book that I enjoy reading and set a timer for fifteen minutes. After fifteen minutes of free reading, I can continue reading or move on to a new task.

Spiritual: I intend to spend more time in peaceful silence with myself. First step: create time on my calendar that signals me to take fifteen minutes of my day to be in silence with myself. I can meditate and focus on my breath.

Your intentions and "first steps" will vary as your life allows. The goal is to set your intentions in writing and follow through with the "first steps". Keep in mind that you can focus on one, or a few intentions, at a time. You get to choose which intentions you need at any particular moment (some days may feel more physical than spiritual and vice versa). Setting intentions and following through with them offers you the opportunity to focus on your needs.

<u>**Affirmation from Angels and Spirit**</u>:

Time for myself is just as valid and important as the time I spend with the loving beings around me. I take time to focus my energies on my own needs and intentions. When I take time to express things that I truly desire and set my intentions, my energies will rise to a higher vibration and allow me to find more peace in my life.

Empathy and Compassion

Empathy is the ability to feel what others are feeling; it is about having the ability to walk in someone else's shoes and know where she is coming from in her experiences and feelings. It is easy to tell someone else, "I know how you feel" and possess a genuine concern for the other person. However, we often do not know how to express this same empathy for *ourselves*.

I remember telling myself to stop sulking and move on with my life with little regard to how I actually felt (sad, angry, weak, vulnerable, in pain, etc.). It is okay to say, "I know how you feel" to *yourself* and to treat yourself as you would another person who is walking in your shoes. You do not need to beat yourself up for being vulnerable and walking in crappy shoes. Think of it as having the ability to validate and empower yourself into knowing that you need to be kind, compassionate, and gentle with YOU.

<u>**"E-Motion" Step- Have Compassion for Yourself**</u>

A question I have learned to ask myself when I feel *yucky* about lupus is, "What would I say to someone if she told me she felt sad/angry/in pain/fatigued, etc....?" I do not usually respond to that question with, "I don't care," or "Go away, I'm busy." Instead, I often ask the other person why she feels the way she feels and then offer an ear to listen and a shoulder to cry on, if needed. I am learning to do this for *myself* as well.

Compassion comes from our hearts and actions and is the stuff that makes us laugh and cry. When we practice compassion, we are truly in the center of how we feel. We experience a sense of kindness, concern, and consideration. It is a step beyond just identifying and *knowing* what we feel – it is demonstrating the ability to express *how* we feel. I am demonstrating compassion when I say, "I know how you feel" and then express that feeling with a positive action - like a hug. For example, if I say to myself, "I feel sad," and then ask for a hug from a family member, a friend, or myself, I am taking positive action. This validates my sadness with a compassionate act. I can hug myself and validate my feelings with compassion.

Take a moment to validate how you *truly* feel and then *validate* that feeling by assuring yourself with, "I know how you feel. It's crappy, right?" Honor this empathy with an act of compassion (e.g., a hug, a good cry, a nap, a walk, eating healthy food). Show empathy, concern, and compassion with *yourself* just as you would another person.

Affirmation from Angels and Spirit:

I am gentle and kind with myself. I validate and offer compassion to all of my feelings and concerns. I embrace how and why I have my feelings and I offer empathy and compassion to myself. I am walking in my own shoes and I validate my feelings with empathy and compassion.

"E-Motion Step"- Show Gratitude

I often create lists of everything for which I am grateful. When I focus specifically on lupus, I am reminded of all the things I am grateful for while managing this condition. Gratitude can be as simple as writing the name of someone while stating you are grateful, or sending blessings to those people and things that make your life easier.

- Doctors – Doctors are people too. Send them blessings that keep them healthy and informed. Send thoughts of gratitude to your doctors. This can also be as simple as saying, "Thank you" the next time you meet with your doctor(s).

- Family, Friends, and Co-Workers– Send blessings to those who help you. Send love and light to everyone who makes your life easier to manage. Send thank you cards (or emails or texts).

- Medications- Envision your medication(s) as Light and feel gratitude for the *positive* effects of the medication(s).

Continue your gratitude list to include everything for which you are grateful.

Affirmation from Angels and Spirit:

I feel gratitude for everything and everyone who guides and helps me while I manage the needs of my body. I send blessings, light, and love to everything and everyone who guides me.

Part 4

Breathing and Keeping Track of Stuff with Spirit as a Guide

Angel Guidance Messages

Two practices I have adopted to help manage the pain and stress of lupus are "Focused Breathing" and a "Journal with an additional Question List for Doctors".

Pain is one of the body's natural responses to foreign stimuli. Our physical bodies are designed to let us know when something is "wrong" by triggering our pain receptors. Lupus causes inflammation, so the body senses that something is always "wrong", and it responds with pain. The most conventional way to manage chronic pain related to lupus is to use medication that reduces inflammation. In addition to medication, I have discovered that when I travel inside (go within) my body, I am better able to manage pain. The book, *The Lupus Book: A Guide for Patients and Their Families* (2004) offers alternative methods such as biofeedback, acupressure, acupuncture, guided imagery and meditation (Wallace, 198) to help reduce pain. I successfully use guided imagery and meditation as additional tools for managing the pain I experience from inflammation.

I frequently facilitate guided visualization meditations for others, and it has taken time for me to learn how to facilitate this process for myself. At its core, meditation is simply the ability to take a moment to "go within" and acknowledge your body, mind, and Spirit without distractions. Common beliefs about meditation such as: it requires a lot of time, you need special instruction, you need to be in a state of Zen, it requires a specific type of breathing, you need to practice it during a specific time of day, etc. can

29

be natural blocks to the practice of meditation. None of these common beliefs needs to be a block while learning the basics of meditation. Meditation is simply taking a moment to acknowledge inner peace without distraction. This sense of peace allows the body to relax. Relaxation = less pain. The following practice is an easy form of mediation designed to help reduce pain.

Practice: Focusing on Breath and White Light

(***NOTE: Please read this practice prior to engaging in it for the first time).

- Find a quiet area of your home, or go to a quiet place outside. Make sure that you will not be distracted for at least five minutes (turn off your cell phone, close your door, turn off any alarms or other devices that can distract you). Ask others to leave you alone for five to ten minutes (or more, if needed).

- Lie on your back or sit up – whichever position is comfortable for you.

- Close your eyes. Take in a slow, very deep breath of air in through your nose. Breathe the air into your belly – feeling the air expand your lungs and belly. Hold for 1-2 seconds and exhale through your mouth. Repeat this breath three (3) or more times until you feel relaxed.

- Inhale again deeply through your nose while you envision White Light entering and filling your entire body.

- Exhale through your mouth and breathe out any pain, frustration, distractions, etc. Let go of anything that is occupying your mind and prevents you from focusing on your breath.

- Inhale White Light and Exhale Pain several times. You can envision certain pain areas in your body and breathe White Light into those specific areas. Exhale the pain from specific areas. Inhale White Light, Exhale Pain.

  Feel free to use any colors of Light that feel comfortable to you (each color resonates at a different frequency and you may feel different energy vibrations based upon the color you choose to use). White Light includes all of the colors, so it is usually the easiest to begin with when you are first learning to practice your breathing.

- When you feel relaxed, envision your entire body surrounded with White Light.

- Open your eyes slowly when you are finished with your breathing and White Light practice. Take a few deep breaths prior to standing.

You may feel warm/cold/tingly/relaxed, etc. - these are all normal responses. Allow your breathing to guide your body toward reducing pain. Feel free to increase/decrease the time you spend focusing on your breathing. Whenever I experience pain during my day and I am not able to "take five minutes of peace", I take a few deep breaths and envision White Light entering my body while I envision pain leaving my body. Your intention to release pain can manifest once you focus on your breath. When our bodies experience pain, it is often a signal to rest, breath, and heal. Take a moment to rest, breathe, and heal.

Angel Guidance Message:

Give yourself time and space to rest and heal. Your body is a magnificent embodiment of your Spirit. Be gentle with your body and allow it to rest. Pain needs love and rest to resolve. Each time you acknowledge the needs of your body, you honor its abilities to heal. Send love to your body and its signals of pain.

Practice: Journal and Question List for Doctors

As most of us know, keeping track of which doctor said/recommended what thing at when time can be challenging even when our bodies feel healthy. Most of my doctors ask similar questions, so I have found it easier to keep track of dates and important information in a simple 4x6 journal that I bring with me to every doctor's appointment.

My journal looks like this:

- Main pages – Keep track of ongoing daily stuff that is "new" or interesting (a flare, fever, ulcer, first day of medication, doctor's appointment notes, etc.). I do not usually need to write in this area every day, but I write in this area when I have something new or interesting to note.

- Sectioned pages (with tabs) to keep track of specific dates. These pages are useful when one of my doctors asks a question like, "How much Prednisone® are you taking now?" (I have a "Prednisone® section"). I have a "bloodletting section" (my pet name for my frequent lab blood work). In my bloodletting section, I write the date and from which arm blood is drawn. I also have a "flare up" section where I write the dates of when my body is experiencing a flare up. Choose which symptoms, medications, dates, etc. are most important to you and create individual sections for them.

- Sticky Notes with Questions for Doctors- Sticky Notes travel with the Main Pages and have the Doctor's name/Specialty written on the top. I can usually email my doctors with pressing questions, but the "can wait" questions stay on traveling Sticky Notes within my journal.

- Doctor's Appointment notes – I take notes during my appointments with my doctors. This way, I am not limited to the "after visit summary" if my doctor makes a new recommendation or orders a new test. These notes also help when one of my doctor's has a recommendation for another doctor (e.g., an additional blood test or x-ray six months from now).

Your brain does not need to store *every* piece of information, and your sections and method of keeping a journal may differ from mine. The goal is to reduce stress by writing down important information for future reference. Try not to make the journal keeping process itself a stressful endeavor – keep it simple and easy for you to follow.

Practical Stuff

Below are a few practical items that I have found useful for managing my journey with lupus. You may also discover new practical methods for managing lupus. Here are a few that work for me:

- The Lupus Foundation of America™ (lupus.org) website has a plethora of resources for the "pragmatic" aspects of managing lupus: disability, balancing home and work, hair loss, research, new treatments, etc. In addition, the website has links to free teleconferences facilitated by doctors.
- Isolation is a common theme among those of us who manage Lupus. Stay "in touch" with friends and family (even if it is just via email, social media, or phone calls). I also find comfort in knowing that my Angels are always with me.

- Keep informed about the status of lupus in your body and act on any changes by seeking medical attention, if needed. The more your medical team knows, the better your treatment may be.

- If needed, read/ join/create blogs, message boards, and other social media tools to stay informed, vent, and exchange information.

- Make sure to have your doctors / care team explain anything you do not understand. I tend to research information I do not know before and after a visit with my team to make sure I am able to keep up with what is happening with my health and treatments.

- An Advanced Healthcare Directive put my mind and soul at ease. Advanced Healthcare Directives are available at most doctor's offices. You usually need to ask your doctor (or receptionist at your doctor's office) for a copy.

- Finding a great Therapist (Psychotherapist) and/or a Lupus Support Group can be a blessing in helping manage Lupus. It is nice to be in a safe environment where you are able to share your emotions and receive support. The Lupus Foundation of America™ (lupus.org) has a "Support" link on their website so you can locate a local lupus chapter in your area.

- If it feels right, share information from lupus-related websites and pages on social media. You are being an advocate by spreading the word.

Final "E-Motion" Step and Affirmation

The Angel and Spirit messages and affirmations in this book have focused on taking care of YOU while managing lupus. This final thought is a summary that encompasses the "big picture" for you and the management of lupus from the love of Spirit.

"E-Motion" Step:

Follow your intuition and your "gut" feelings about yourself and your life. You are a beautiful Soul who lives in an amazing body, so you are the one who knows what you need (when you take time to ask yourself what you need). Be kind and gentle with yourself and follow through with what your body needs. Show empathy, compassion, and love for yourself at all times.

Affirmation from Angels and Spirit:

I am a beautiful Soul and I live in an amazing body. I will ask my body what it needs, and I will be kind, gentle, and show empathy to myself. I will offer myself compassion and love at all times.

Many blessings as you travel with your Amazing Mind, Body and Spirit

Quick "Pick Me Up" Affirmations

- *I am a Being of Love and Light. I radiate Unconditional Love and Light to others and myself.*

- *It is safe for me to let go of guilt and stress. My body will let me know when it needs rest and I honor my body's need for rest without feelings of guilt or stress.*

- *My body is beautiful. I honor my body without judgement.*

- *I ask my body, "What do I need today?" and follow through with these needs.*

- *I have empathy and compassion for myself. I hold myself in the highest esteem.*

- *I envision Light and Love surrounding my body at all times.*

- *I am walking in my own shoes and I validate my feelings with empathy and compassion.*

- *I advocate my needs at all times.*

- *I ask for help. By doing so, I honor the compassion and love of another.*

- *My needs and desires are valid. I take time to create and affirm my intentions each day.*

- *My Guardian Angels and Angels surround me at all times. I am never alone.*

- *I am gentle with myself.*

- *When I radiate from Spirit, I radiate love.*

- *I focus on my breath and envision pain leaving my body. I take time to rest, breathe, and heal.*

- *I feel gratitude for everything and everyone who guides and helps me while I manage the needs of my body. I send blessings, light, and love to everything and everyone who guides me.*

- *I speak up for myself freely and easily. I claim my own power. I love and approve of myself. I am free and safe"* (Hay, p. 184).

Works Cited

Daniel J. Wallace, M. (2009). *The Lupus Book 4th Edition.* New York: Oxford University Press.

Hay, L. L. (2004). *You Can Heal Your Life.* Carlsbad: Hay House, Inc. hayhouse.com

Lupus Foundation of America™ Walk to End Lupus Now®. *lupus.org.* (2014)., Inc.: www.lupus.org. http://www.lupus.org/page/-/files/pdf/Lupus_Factsheet.pdf

Lupus Foundation of America™. lupus.org. (2014, May 25)..

Virtue, D. (2011). *The Angel Therapy Handbook.* Carlsbad: Hay House, Inc. hayhouse.com

Virtue, D. and The Angelic Realm. (1997). *Angel Therapy: Healing Messages for Every Area of Your Life.* Carlsbad: Hay House, Inc. hayhouse.com.

Recommended Reading

- Hollingsworth, C. (2013). *Reconnecting with Your TRUE Self: Easy and To-the-Point Guidance for Remembering Your Connection with Your Spirit.* Amazon.com. http://www.amazon.com/Reconnecting-Your-TRUE-Self-point/dp/1493581473/ref=cm_sw_em_r_dp_6Vj1sb1Y5MNKss42_lm

- Lupus Foundation of America™. *Lupus Now* magazine. Washington, D.C. lupusnow.org.

- McNamara, L. RN & Kemper, K. PhD (2011). *If You Have to Wear an Ugly Dress, Learn to Accessorize: Guidance, Inspiration, and Hope for Women with Lupus, Scleroderma, and Other Autoimmune Illnesses.* Tucson: Wheatmark®.

- Price, J.R. (1987). *The Abundance Book.* Carlsbad: Hay House, Inc. hayhouse.com.

- Stein, D. (2004). *The Women's Book of Healing.* Berkeley, CA: The Crossing Press. www.tenspeed.com.

- Weed, Susan S. (2002). *The New Menopausal Years: The Wise Woman Way Alternative Approaches for Women 30-90.* Woodstock, NY: Ash Tree Publishing.

Recommended Websites

- Alf.org: Alliance for Lupus Research (ALR).

- Angeltherapy.com. Doreen Virtue.

- Arthritis.org: The Arthritis Foundation.

- Lupus.org. Lupus Foundation of America™.

- Christine Miserandino: www.butyoudontlooksick.com/category/the-**spoon-theory**/

by Christine Miserandino www.butyoudontlooksick.com - See more at:

http://www.butyoudontlooksick.com/articles/written-by-christine/the-spoon-

theory/#sthash.mFiio1Yf.dpuf

- Unity.org. Association of Unity Churches.

Recommended DVD

- Lam, P. Dr. (2009). *Tai Chi for Arthritis*. Tai Chi Productions.
  www.taichiproductions.com.

- Lupus Foundation of America™. (2004). *The Right Moves For Lupus*: A Gentle Fitness
  Program. Piedmont Chapter. www.lupuslinks.org. 704.375.8787.

About the Author

Cory Hollingsworth is a Certified Angel Therapy Practitioner® and Spiritual Medium.

Cory has been working with the Angelic Realm since 2001 and has guided

hundreds of people with their journeys of Self-Discovery and Intuition.

Cory facilitates Angel Readings, Workshops, and HeartLight Seminars throughout the

United States and is guided to help others to remember their Connection with their

Higher Self and their own Intuitive Gifts. By connecting with YOUR HIGHER SELF and

YOUR SPIRIT GUIDES, Cory offers guidance and insights into your Life Purposes, Soul

Contracts, and Life Lessons.

Cory is also the author of the book *Reconnecting with Your TRUE Self: Easy and To-*

The-Point Guidance for Remembering Your Connection with Your Spirit.

Cory has appeared on the television program *Paranormal Connection* and on the radio

show *Psychic Talk*. She is also the Co-Founder of *HeartLight Energy Seminars*.

Visit Cory's Websites: http://coryangeldragonfly.wix.com/coryhollingsworth

Facebook: Cory Angel Hollingsworth

Author photo courtesy of Paula Watson at Planet Earth Rising

Planetearthrising.com

DISCLAIMER

The guidance and advice from the author does not offer a prescription, a promise of benefits, claims of cures, or a guarantee of results.

The information, instruction or advice given by the author/practitioner is not intended to be a substitute for competent professional medical or psychological diagnosis and care.

Do not discontinue or modify any medication presently being taken pursuant to medical advice without obtaining approval from your healthcare professional.

NOTE: The "Little Lupus Book: Blending the Facts about Lupus with Spirit" was originally intended to be printed in a 4x6 inch format, hence making it "little". Due to formatting "issues" and the author's impatience with "messing with" margins, the "little" book remained in its original 8.5x11 inch format. In addition, this size is easier to hold with hands that are experiencing pain. It is also easier to "flatten out" while simultaneously reading and meditating.

www.ingramcontent.com/pod-product-compliance
Lightning Source LLC
Chambersburg PA
CBHW081536280526
45788CB00010B/3254